RECENT ADVANCES IN
MEDICAL SCIENCE

*A Study of their Social and
Economic Implications*

RECENT ADVANCES IN
MEDICAL SCIENCE

*A Study of their Social and
Economic Implications*

by

SIR EDWARD MELLANBY

K.C.B., M.D., F.R.C.P., F.R.S., K.H.P.

Secretary to the Medical Research Council

THE REDE LECTURE
DELIVERED BEFORE THE UNIVERSITY
OF CAMBRIDGE ON 28 APRIL 1939

CAMBRIDGE

AT THE UNIVERSITY PRESS

1939

CAMBRIDGE
UNIVERSITY PRESS

University Printing House, Cambridge CB2 8BS, United Kingdom

Published in the United States of America by Cambridge University Press, New York

Cambridge University Press is part of the University of Cambridge.

It furthers the University's mission by disseminating knowledge in the pursuit of education, learning and research at the highest international levels of excellence.

www.cambridge.org
Information on this title: www.cambridge.org/9781107637078

© Cambridge University Press 1939

First published 1939
First paperback edition 2014

A catalogue record for this publication is available from the British Library

ISBN 978-1-107-63707-8 Paperback

Recent Advances in Medical Science
A Study of their Social and
Economic Implications

Probably at no time in the world's history has the
average citizen of this and of most other civilised
communities felt so insecure against death by
violence. At no time in the world's history has
the same citizen had reason to feel so secure against
death by disease.

The cause of the first of these outlooks fills us
with despair: the cause of the second gives us great
satisfaction. It seemed opportune, therefore, that
this year's Robert Rede lecture should be devoted
to an account of certain of man's activities which
have formed the basis of his present-day sense of
security of health. It may be possible by this means,
at a time when many are doubting whether sanity
and righteousness occupy the dominant place
usually ascribed to them, to restore to their minds
a firmer belief in the power of the human intellect
to guide their destiny. If war and present-day
national policy in many countries are based on the
assumption that human life is nothing, except in
so far as it contributes to national power, the basis
of my discourse to-day is different, namely, that
human life and health, developed and enjoyed to

a maximum degree by each individual, are in themselves the most precious of all things in the world.

The mind of man has never been so active as it has been during the turmoil of recent years in analysing social, economic and political factors in the endeavour to appraise the part played by each in national and international existence. In these analyses one of the greatest revolutionary changes, which has influenced the life of almost every individual in civilised communities, has been generally overlooked, both by the public and even by the leaders of sociology and history. I refer to the effects of the rapid advance of knowledge in medical science. This knowledge has brought to mankind the means of conquering many diseases, of improving the standard of health and physique of the average individual to a degree never known before and of warding off death itself. This kind of victory of the human mind is wholly and universally beneficial to the individual, and has not been obtained by one race at the expense of another, but by the finest type of international co-operation. It represents one of the highest intellectual efforts ever made and, by reducing pain, suffering and grief, on the one hand, and by increasing the benefits of life and the power of appreciation of much that is best in it on the other hand, has contributed greatly to the advance in human happiness and efficiency. Its success represents a vast achievement, and its certain promise of even greater success in the future cannot but act as an antidote to the present political insanity of the world.

My theme to-day is not to be confined to the singing of a pæan of praise centring round these modern advances in knowledge and the control they bring over human suffering, but it is also to call attention to some of the social and economic implications of such knowledge. Some of these effects, which I can only briefly mention in the course of a lecture, are clearly of great importance and require the attention of others more highly qualified than myself. Lowered mortality rates, longer life and improved standards of health and physique must be factors of prime importance in all aspects of national and international life, and since, short of a world catastrophe, all these changes are likely to increase greatly in the future, it may be wise for students of mankind to consider now their probable influence on the community and on the world in general in years to come. Whereas most individuals will interpret these developments as beneficial to themselves and their families, it is certain that, from the point of view of the State, some may not be beneficial but even, in certain respects, harmful. No subject can less afford to be dealt with by emotional, uninformed and haphazard methods; only by knowledge and careful foresight can the best be made of the great advances in the conquest of disease.

Many people do not appreciate what a frail thing human life, especially early life, is, and what a small chance there was for the average baby to survive, until medical science entered the field. Less than 200 years ago, i.e. up to the year 1750, 74 per cent of all children born in London died before reaching the age of five. At present, probably less than 12 per cent of all children born in this country die before reaching this age. Thus, in spite of a great decrease in the fertility rate of women and much emigration, a population, stationary for many centuries, was changed to the rapidly expanding one of the past century. You will, therefore, realise why it can be claimed with reason that medical science, by placing in the hands of man powerful weapons for combating disease, may be regarded as the greatest practical factor that has influenced human society. Parenthetically I may add that, in view of these and other facts to be mentioned, it is often a cause of amazement to see the low esteem in which many people hold medical science, although this seldom extends to their private medical practitioners. If there is any doubt on this matter, the perusal of a discussion in the House of Commons on any health topic will quickly confirm this statement.

THE ADOPTION OF THE EXPERIMENTAL
METHOD IN MEDICAL INVESTIGATION

It is unnecessary before my present audience to dwell on the reasons why medical science has made such great progress, especially in the last sixty years. It followed immediately on the realisation that the experimental method is the royal road to discovery, not only in the case of inanimate matter but also in relation to the structure, functions and diseases of organisms, including man himself. When he was faced with the limitation of experimenting on man, the scientist came to appreciate the great potentialities of investigating the reactions of lower forms of life, and he seized this opportunity with both hands. Occasionally, in attempting to extend the newly discovered facts of biology to man, he has been wrong but, generally speaking, this weapon of research has proved of immense value in terms both of human and animal life and health. With the acceptance of the modern view that medicine is a scientific study, that disease need not be associated with ideas of guilt or superstition or that it has supernatural implications, that health is the normal state and a right of man, all the older views of ill-health, which have lasted throughout the ages and which were based mainly on religious teachings, have been superseded. Man has at last been able to get down to the study of actual disease and has wrested from nature sufficient facts greatly to extend the control of his own destiny.

Even during this period of advance of knowledge, the attitude of medical science towards its problems has changed rapidly. In the first period of expansion, following the work of Pasteur, Lister and Koch, there was a tendency to regard all disease as due to the invasion of the body by some form of micro-organism. This hypothesis led to a wonderful advance in the control of many diseases. It then became clear that other diseases could not be explained on this basis and that much ill-health was due to some chemical abnormality in the body, the lack or excess of some substance which upset the balance necessary for health. Sometimes this unbalance was due to wrong diet, providing too little or too much of certain chemical factors, sometimes the failure was more attributable to defective working of certain body cells themselves, and the whole subject of hormonic disharmony was revealed. In more recent years it has become evident that invasion of the body by pathogenic micro-organisms and lack of chemical balance of the body are often associated, and even that the pathogenicity of micro-organisms is itself a chemical problem. We have now arrived at the stage when the human body, from the point of view of health and disease, has become largely a problem of co-ordinated and balanced chemical reactions, and investigations are directed more and more to the study of chemical changes compatible and incompatible with the proper functioning of tissues. Once a biological observation has been made, be it physiological, pathological or clinical (and biological discoveries are always the most difficult to make in medical science), the investigator of the present day knows that the observed phenomenon will be extended and interpreted in terms of chemistry. It is this hypothesis and the sense of certainty it conveys that accounts for much of the success and optimism of the modern investigator in medical science.

ADVANCES IN THE CONTROL OF HUMAN DISEASE

While the physiologist and pathologist have been patiently building up the foundation of knowledge of the body in health and disease and providing the basis upon which all advancement in medical science depends, others have investigated the more applied side of curative and preventive medicine. The immunologist has taught mankind how to control, either by prevention or cure, many infective diseases by inoculation with toxins, toxoids and antitoxins, vaccines and antisera. Increased control has thus been obtained over diphtheria, measles, whooping cough, cerebrospinal fever, tetanus and anthrax. The extension of physiology and biochemistry, even in the last twenty-five years, has opened up the field of nutritional disease and thereby provided control of such conditions as rickets, osteomalacia, defective tooth formation, scurvy, beri-beri, pellagra and night blindness, and also revolutionised the most important subject of feeding, especially of infants and growing children.

Since antipyrin, acetanilide and phenacetin were prepared in the laboratory and prescribed for the relief of pain fifty years ago, the use of synthetic drugs for the treatment of symptoms and indeed for the actual cure of disease has achieved great success. The introduction of organic arsenicals by Ehrlich in 1910 for the cure of syphilis was followed by the discovery of other synthetic drugs for the cure of malaria, bilharzia, kala azar and sleeping sickness. In the past three years we have seen the wonderful effects of another type of chemotherapeutic agent, namely, the sulphanilamide derivatives which, from the point of view of disease in this country, probably represent the greatest advance in treatment of the present century. Until these discoveries were made, no instance of a chemotherapeutic agent having a specific effect on bacterial infections was known. Now streptococcal, meningococcal and pneumococcal infections, previously the most deadly of all diseases, have for the most part been brought under control. Sepsis and septicaemia of child-birth, meningitis, erysipelas, gonorrhoea and in-fections of the genito-urinary tract and pneumonia are now treated successfully with such drugs as prontosil, sulphanilamide and the more recently discovered 2-sulphanilyl-aminopyridine. In the past month it was reported that, in a series of between 600 and 700 cases of pneumonia at Bir-mingham, the mortality rate was lowered, in the case of patients under fifty years of age, from 17 to 1·6 per cent and in patients over fifty years, from 50 to 24 per cent by the use of 2-sulphanilyl-aminopyridine (W. F. Gaisford, *Lancet*, 1939, 1, 823). In observations made in the Sudan, the mortality rate of cerebrospinal fever was reduced from one varying between 70 and 95 per cent to 5 per cent by the use of these drugs.

Before leaving this subject of disease control, it is also necessary to refer in passing to the triumphs of recent work on hormones—to the modern methods of treating diabetes mellitus with insulin, pernicious anaemia with liver active principle, Addison's disease with substances prepared from the adrenal cortex, myxoedema with thyroxine, and various conditions amenable to treatment by sex hormones. This is also one of the most active divisions of medical science.

For brevity's sake it is only possible to recount

(13)

here a few of the triumphs of modern medical research. These are the fruits of the tree, the tree itself being, from a scientific point of view, vastly more important than its fruit. May I also add that in this amazing growth there are no more active branches in the world than are found in the medical school of this university?

As for other outstanding examples of the effects on health and disease in man of the application of increments of knowledge, these can be cited briefly. The adoption of better standards of sanitation and cleanliness, developed and supported by the science of bacteriology and immunology, cleared out of the country many of the decimating diseases of past centuries. Plague, malaria, typhus, cholera and smallpox, which killed their thousands and tens of thousands, disappeared in the nineteenth century. Typhoid fever which, even in the year 1900 killed over 5000 people in this country, was responsible for the death of only 206 people in 1937, and any mild epidemic nowadays is liable to create a great public scandal.

Other infectious diseases, although still with us, have been reduced greatly in their killing power. Tuberculosis, which in the years 1871–80 killed annually in this country 2880 out of every 100,000 people, had a mortality rate of 690 only in 1937. Mortality due to scarlet fever sank from 720 per 100,000 people in the years 1871–80 to 9 in 1937.

The corresponding figures for measles were 380 in 1871–80 and 26 in 1937; for whooping cough 510 in 1871–80 and 43 in 1937. These are some of the main fatal diseases in childhood, and it is on human life at this age that medical science has had its greatest influence.

Infant mortality has fallen in the last forty years from 156 per 1000 to 53 per 1000, but the corresponding figure of 31 per 1000 for New Zealand still indicates plenty of room for improvement. How great has been the change in childhood and early adult life can be understood from the fact that, whereas even so short a time ago as 1922, 42·5 per cent of all deaths in Britain occurred before the age of fifty, and 57·5 per cent after fifty, in 1937 only 27 per cent of deaths occurred under fifty and 73 per cent after this age.

With the shrinkage of the death-rate in early life, the rapid raising of the average age of the population and the postponement of death, there has been, as might be expected, an increased incidence in the fatal diseases of later life and probably an increase in the disabling and degenerative diseases associated with advancing years. As regards the former, the increase in mortality due to diseases of the heart and circulation has been exceptionally great in the present century. In 1935 the mortality rate due to heart disease was more than five times greater in this country than in

1921. As regards death due to angina pectoris, there was an increase amounting to 176 per cent in males and 206 per cent in females over the corresponding figures even such a short time ago as 1928. Apart from any differences in these figures that may be accounted for by differences of diagnosis or in age distribution, there is a strong suggestion that some harmful cause of heart disease and especially of coronary occlusion, probably some mistake in mode of living, has recently appeared in our midst or has become accentuated. This matter urgently needs attention by scientists.

As might be expected, deaths due to cancer have risen in recent years, the crude mortality rate having increased from 1336 per million living in 1925 to 1633 in 1937. Taking the crude mortality rate at 100 in 1901–10, the corresponding figure in 1935 was 204 among males and 155 among females. In view of the great difference in age distribution between these years, the increase is not surprising, and there is not much support for the view that cancer has increased more rapidly than can be accounted for by the large number of older people now living.

Were the effects of eliminating the mortal diseases of early life, which thereby postpone death, the only claims of medical science, they would be sufficiently large. But much more than this can be claimed for it. Almost as important is its effect on the quality of life and the general advance in physique and health of the population. Especially can this be seen in the physique of school boys and girls. In the twenty years, 1911–31, the average height and weight of boys of twelve years of age attending elementary schools in Leeds increased from 4 ft. 4 in. and 63·5 lb. to 4 ft. 7 in. and 74·4 lb. respectively. Sir Henry Bashford reports similar changes among those employed at the Post Office, the present-day boys aged sixteen being 16 lb. heavier and 1½ in. taller than boys of the same age twenty-five years ago: girls of sixteen are 10 lb. heavier on an average and 1 in. taller than girls of the same age of the last generation. Most or all of these improvements in physique are now known to be due to changes in food habits, and to the increased consumption of the protective foods—milk, butter, eggs, fruit and vegetables—at the expense of bread and other cereals.

In addition to the improved height and weight, there has also been a great decrease in bone deformity in young people. Bandy legs in children, which used to be a matter of indifference or amusement, are now rare and their occurrence gives rise to feelings of indignation. Even in north-country towns, where rickets used to be a veritable plague, the reduction in its incidence has been very great, and cases are often difficult to find for teaching purposes. The decrease in bone and glandular tuberculosis has also been remarkable.

Probably sufficient has been said to indicate the nature and degree of decrease in disease and the improvement in health and physique made possible by the application of medical science in recent years.

MEDICAL DISCOVERY AND SOCIAL LIFE

But it may be objected that most of the great improvements in health and the reduction in mortality are not due primarily to new knowledge gained through medical research but to administrative actions of government and local government, such as the introduction of drainage, removal of refuse, pure water supplies and attention to the purity of food. Moderation in the use of alcoholic beverages and better habits of personal cleanliness and outdoor recreation will also be assigned important places in the improvement of standards of health. The part played by these changes in mode of living is, of course, inestimably great, but all of them represent changes either based entirely upon scientific discovery of the cause of disease or strongly supported and sanctioned by such discovery. Scientific knowledge of the causation or control of disease is, of course, quite fruitless unless it is practically applied either by governing authorities, by doctors or by individuals. At the

(18)

same time, as I shall show later, the success of administration and public action in combating disease is limited by the knowledge made available by scientific investigation.

Some changes in the mode of living become so ingrained in the people as social habits that their origin is often forgotten. Probably the best example of this is seen in the modern habit of personal cleanliness, which has become a measure almost of aestheticism and social standing. But surely the primary stimulus to personal cleanliness of the present day is almost entirely the knowledge of bacteriology and its offspring infection. A good example of the effect of official action towards a greater cleanliness is seen in the case of the children of the London County Council schools, which is no doubt typical of most schools of the same kind in the country. In 1912, 39·5 per cent of these children had parasitic skin infections. Greater cleanliness was insisted upon by the authorities, with the result that by 1920 this percentage was reduced to 13·8, in 1934 to 4·5, and in 1937 to 2·6. Ringworm of the scalp was formerly one of the greatest scourges of school children. In these same schools in 1911 there were 6214 new cases of this disease, in 1920 there were 3983, in 1934 265 and in 1937 only 78. Many other instances of the same kind could be given, but these examples will probably suffice to show that personal cleanliness,

(19)

as at present practised, is not an ingrained instinct, as many seem to think, but is largely the outcome of a public effort based on the knowledge acquired by medical investigation that many infective diseases of mankind are dirt diseases. Nor must we forget the part played in this crusade by those who manufacture and sell soap.

If there is still doubt as to the power of science in relation to diseases of uncleanliness in the bacteriological sense, it is only necessary to study the story of the detection of the two persons who were the origins of the recent outbreaks of typhoid fever at Bournemouth and Croydon respectively. Neither of these men at the time of his detection had any idea that he harboured the typhoid micro-organism in his alimentary canal. Similarly, the modern method of tracking down individuals who have transmitted certain types of streptococci, often from their throats, to women in childbirth represents scientific detection at its best.

The scientist engaged in medical research will not complain of the basis assigned for public and private changes in habits of living which have proved so beneficial to health. What he does complain of is the great delay which often occurs before many of the teachings, which his investigations have elucidated, are adopted by public authorities and private citizens. In some cases the absence of application is due to administrative inertia or to lack of political and social interest, in some to ignorance or laziness on the part of the public, and more often it is due to such economic and social restrictions as prevent people from attaining the nutritional and hygienic conditions necessary for healthy existence. The medical scientist knows, for instance, that diphtheria could be cleared out of this country at once by the preventive inoculation of infants and children by diphtheria toxoid. He has seen this happen in the state of Ontario in Canada. In the town of Hamilton, Ontario, with a population of 155,000, not one case of diphtheria has been diagnosed in the past five years. In the city of Quebec, on the other hand, where prophylaxis by inoculation of diphtheria toxoid was not used, the deaths from diphtheria in 1936 were even more numerous than in 1927. In New York City he has seen a reduction in diphtheria incidence from 8548 cases in 1929 to 1143 in 1936, and a reduction in deaths from 463 to 35 following the introduction of preventive inoculation. In this country diphtheria is still the commonest single cause of death among school children. In 1937 there were 61,339 cases of this disease in England and Wales causing 2963 deaths, mostly in children between the ages of one and fifteen years. Apart from these unnecessary family tragedies, think of the public expense involved. The average child with diphtheria stays about six weeks in a public fever hospital. Assuming that the cost per week for nursing, treatment and maintenance is about £4, it will be seen that the direct cost to the country of this disease is of the order of £1,500,000 annually. When the medical scientist thinks of an instance like this, where his work has gone largely disregarded for ten years or more, he feels in despair.

An even better example, although in this case social and economic conditions make the application of knowledge more difficult, is seen in the field of nutrition. Every expert in this field knows that the consumption of proper food from birth onwards would revolutionise the standards of physique and health. He sees enormous differences in the physique of the poor as compared with that of the well-to-do. For instance, the average height and weight of boys at the age of eleven attending a better-class school are 55·33 in. and 76·22 lb. respectively, while the corresponding figures for elementary school boys of the same age are 3 in. and 12 lb. less respectively. He sees also the great difference in the death-rate of children of the poor as compared with that of the children of the well-to-do. The following tables illustrate this point by giving the mortality rates of children up to one year and between one and two years, classified according to the social status of the father.

Table I

Rates per 100,000 legitimate live births for deaths under 1 year

	All	I	II	III	IV	V
Premature birth	1730	1050	1440	1680	1860	1960
Injury at birth	210	230	250	210	200	200
Congenital malformations	550	500	540	560	570	540
Congenital debility	300	140	220	290	330	380
Infantile convulsions	210	130	170	200	260	230
Whooping cough	180	30	100	160	210	270
Tuberculosis, all forms	100	30	60	90	110	130
Bronchitis and pneumonia	1270	280	610	1120	1450	1880
Diarrhoea and enteritis	520	200	260	460	540	790
Accident	80	60	80	70	90	100
Total	5150	2650	3730	4840	5620	6480

Table II

Rates for deaths per 100,000 legitimate children at ages 1–2

	All	I	II	III	IV	V
Measles	242	25	70	194	246	469
Whooping cough	127	28	52	109	140	209
Diphtheria	36	13	18	32	38	55
Tuberculosis, all forms	113	69	73	104	125	150
Influenza	28	16	23	26	24	39
Bronchitis and pneumonia	529	128	223	448	607	861
Diarrhoea and enteritis	72	28	40	60	76	118
Accident	53	19	39	48	56	70
Other causes	252	128	190	237	261	327
Total	1452	454	728	1258	1573	2298

(In the tables, Class I represents the professional and generally well-to-do section of the population, Class III skilled artisan and analogous workers, and Class V labourers and other unskilled callings, while Classes II and IV are intermediates comprising occupations of mixed types or types not readily assignable to the classes on either side.)

Some of the differences in the mortality rates are most impressive. It will be seen, for instance, that the mortality rate due to tuberculosis under the age of one is four times as great in the children of the poorest people as in those of the well-to-do, and between one and two years twice as great. As regards bronchitis and pneumonia, the rate of death in the poorest class is more than six times as great as that among the well-to-do for infants under the age of one, and seven times as great for children of one to two years. In the case of diarrhoea and enteritis there is also a very great discrepancy, the mortality of the poorest children being four times as great as that of the well-to-do children up to the age of two. Altogether it will be seen that, whereas only 2650 per 100,000 legitimate children under the age of one and 454 per 100,000 aged one to two years died in the year 1930–2 among the well-to-do, among the poorest class these figures were raised to 6480 and 2298 respectively. These differences alone will show that we still have a long way to go before we bring down the mortality rate of the poorest children to the figure of the well-to-do children. The day will probably come when the country will regard it as intolerable that the number of deaths of children under two is related to the amount of money received per week by the father of the family. Although these death-rates only refer to children under two years of age, the greater death-rates in the case of some of the diseases such as tuberculosis, bronchitis and pneumonia continue throughout life among the poorer people. Apart from the higher death-rates, statistical records of the distribution of chronic ill-health among the working-class population are very enlightening and help to give some idea of the general situation. The following results were obtained from an analysis made by the Department of Health for Scotland. The total volume of incapacity due to ill-health in the year 1936-7 among the insured population in Scotland was nearly 27 million days or an average of 14·9 days per insured person, and careful analysis shows that there was a constant increase in chronic sickness after the year 1930-1. These figures, at first sight, would convey the impression that there is a tremendous amount of ill-health in the insured people of Scotland. When examined more closely, however, it is found that in the year under review 30,754 persons were continuously incapacitated over the whole twelve months, thus contributing 11,225,000 days to the total sickness experienced. In other words 1·7 per cent only of the insured population, or roughly one in every sixty, accounted for 40 per cent of the 27 million days lost through sickness. In the report it is shown that the number of new cases of chronic incapacity arising in a year bears some relation to the economic conditions prevailing, and that for men under thirty-five years of age tuberculosis and mental diseases accounted for half the total cases, while at later ages bronchitis, pneumonia and rheumatism play an increasing part. Such a large amount of chronic invalidism leads in one sense to too gloomy a picture of the health of the whole insured population. To put it in better perspective, a special sampling enquiry was embarked upon to discover what number of persons had no sickness at all during the year. The answer is very interesting, namely, that 74·8 per cent were never ill, even in a year of widespread influenza, 23·5 per cent were ill on one or more occasions, and the remaining 1·7 per cent already referred to were continuously incapacitated. Thus we see that, in a country like Scotland, chronic ill-health sufficient to bring about complete in-capacitation for work affects only a small propor-tion of the population, although the gross figures in themselves would give the impression of an enormous amount of ill-health.

The same kind of differences between standards of health, which can be tracked down to dietetic and hygienic conditions, are seen in the comparative mortality rates of town and country, although these differences are rapidly disappearing. In the years 1911–14 the average excess of mortality of county boroughs over rural areas was 46 per cent. Twenty years later the average standardised death-rate of the county boroughs had fallen by 31 per cent, that of the other urban areas by 25 per cent, and that of rural areas by 20 per cent, so that the excess of county borough over rural mortality was thus reduced to 25 per cent from the 46 per cent in 1911–14. Generally speaking, it can be said that the more rapid reduction in urban than in rural mortality during recent years shows that the handicap to health imposed by the nutritional and hygienic conditions of urban residence is now little more than half as great as it was a quarter of a century ago.

It is undoubted that the major cause of the differences in physique, standards of health and mortality rates between the different classes of people is nutritional, although there are certainly other hygienic causes. The poorer the people, the more dependent are they on the cheaper foods, and the greater the consumption of bread and other cereals, sugar, jam, lard, margarine and tea, and the less the consumption of the protective dairy and market-gardening products such as milk, eggs, vegetables and fruit. The interaction between poverty, ill-health, defective nutrition and hygiene is cumulative in its effect. Poor people can only afford poor food, they become ill, can earn less money, eat poorer diets and become more ill.

It must be admitted, however, that great improvement has taken place in the dietary of the country during the past twenty years, but there is still room for much further improvement. Since 1909 there has been an increased consumption of 88 per cent in the case of fruit, 64 per cent in vegetables other than potatoes and about 50 per cent in butter and eggs. With the larger consumption of these and other foods, the demand for bread per individual has dropped nearly half in the last century. If the consumption of milk ever shows the same increase as the other protective foods enumerated, the physique and health of the country will again improve very greatly. The present high price, the opposition of many farmers to pasteurisation, and the absence, until recently, of any general effort to supply a clean and bacteriologically safe product have prevented any great increase in the consumption of milk.

It may be that economic and other considerations will prevent fuller advantage being taken of modern teachings on nutrition without much greater government help. It may be that ulti-

(29)

mately the State will guarantee the provision of a sufficiency of protective foods to all school children. This would be a profitable action and the cost of the provision of such food would probably be saved by the diminished cost of medical services and the increased efficiency of the people. It may be that social customs, fashions and taboos will ultimately come to exert an influence in feeding habits as they have done in those of cleanliness. It may happen, for instance, that to give tea to children instead of milk may come to be regarded as bad form, just as it is now considered bad form for people to have unwashed ears.

It will be evident from the instances given previously that, although great improvement in the standard of health has followed the application of knowledge gained by medical research, there is still much ill-health and subnormal development that could be eliminated, if the knowledge at present available were fully used, especially in the case of poor people.

Whereas these statements about the relation of poverty to ill-health are only too true, it would be a mistake if I left the impression that poverty increases the incidence of *all* diseases. It is equally certain that some diseases are much more common among the well-to-do than among the poor. For instance, well-to-do people are much more likely to develop and die of diabetes mellitus, angina pectoris, appendicitis and cirrhosis of the liver than poor people. These diseases might possibly be regarded as diseases of over-indulgence but, except in the case of cirrhosis of the liver, little or nothing is known as to the particular indulgence responsible for each condition. Unlike the commoner diseases among the poor, which act and kill particularly in early life, the diseases of indulgence become more prominent in late adult life. With the increase in the standard of living diabetes mellitus, angina pectoris and appendicitis are becoming more frequent and will probably continue so to do, until medical science has discovered the particular mistakes in the mode of living of those with more money to spend upon themselves.

EFFECTS OF MEDICAL SCIENCE ON HOSPITAL AND OTHER PRACTICE

Discoveries in medical science have had and are having two opposing effects on hospitals and medical practice. On the one side, advances in the diagnosis and treatment of disease, acting in association with a great increase in the social conscience and the greater individual regard for health, have resulted in a need for more hospital accommodation. New methods of diagnosis and treatment, often difficult and costly in time and money, have been discovered. In particular, the technique and skill required in diagnosis by X-ray methods have been improved and extended and the departments concerned with such methods in hospitals have expanded. Similarly, the importance of the clinical laboratory has continually increased, and the services of the bacteriologist, pathologist, biochemist and haematologist are more and more called upon. The developments of modern surgery, with greater control of sepsis, better and safer methods of anaesthesia and improved means of preventing and combating shock, have extended the use of this branch of medicine. All these developments, with their technical requirements, have made it more and more impossible for the sick to get the best attention unless they enter some public institution. No longer are the patients of voluntary hospitals confined to the 'sick poor', and classes of society who, at one time, would not have entered a hospital, now do so with eagerness, paying according to their means, either as patients in general wards or in specially provided pay-beds.

With the introduction of the improved methods of diagnosis and treatment, the cost of hospitals has increased enormously. Professor Johnstone, Superintendent of Guy's Hospital, informs me that, whereas the cost of maintaining a patient for a week in that hospital from 1907 until the war was never less than £1. 18s. 5d. and not more than

£2. 2s. 2d. during the war and the immediate post-war period, there was a steady rise and by 1920 the cost had reached £4. 7s. 8d. and remained fairly constant till 1928 when it reached £4. 11s. 7d. It was again constant for five years, but since 1933 there has been a steady increase and in 1938 it reached the highest point, viz. £5. 16s. 3d. When it is added that in this case there is no charge included for medical and surgical attendance, it will be realised how enormous is the expense of the care of the sick in hospital at the present time. Those who enter hospitals as paying patients will also understand the high charges made for their treatment. It is indeed clear that the future existence of the voluntary hospitals must in many cases be in great jeopardy, especially if the present rate of development continues. It will be observed also that this increase in cost and extent of hospital services does not depend on any actual increase of sickness.

This, however, is only one side of the story. Alongside the great advances in methods of diagnosing and treating disease, another kind of knowledge is accumulating which, by leading to its prevention, is having a diametrically opposite effect on hospital and medical practice. By eliminating disease it makes hospitals, doctors and nursing less necessary. Much less is heard of this kind of discovery, because there is nothing so dramatic about it as there is in the discovery of curative methods which virtually restore patients from the point of death to health. Indeed, the very measure of success of discoveries in preventive medicine is forgetfulness—diseases which are here to-day are gone to-morrow and all the pain, suffering and tragedy associated with them are forgotten.

It might be thought, in view of the great increase in hospital work in recent times, that knowledge of preventive medicine is of negligible importance. This is not, or ought not to be the case. The difficulty is that, whereas curative methods of treatment are immediately taken up, not only in hospitals but also in private practice, prevention of disease is never regarded as a matter of urgency and its adoption is therefore slow. However slow it may be, its action in the end is certain and enduring, and there can be but little doubt that, in the near future, the elimination and reduction of disease by prevention will entirely alter the character of hospital practice, and may indeed greatly reduce the need for institutional treatment. We have seen in our own time the elimination or great reduction in incidence of a number of diseases which, not so long ago, infested our hospitals— rickets, cirrhosis of the liver, summer diarrhoea and vomiting, tuberculosis of glands of the neck and of bones, chlorosis, acute osteomyelitis, scabies,

(34)

ringworm and trachoma—and the list will undoubtedly be substantially increased in the near
future. Rheumatic fever in childhood, one of the
most disabling of all diseases, the aftermath of
which used to be so commonly seen as valvular
disease of the heart of adult life in hospitals, is
rapidly diminishing, at least in the south of England. In 1926, 2 per cent of the London County
Council school children suffered from acquired
heart disease due to acute rheumatism. In 1936
this number had decreased to 0·8 per cent. Cases
of fracture of bones, which occupy so much of
our hospital work, could be diminished at once,
as soon as it is recognised that the bones of most
people in this country are badly formed and that
they can be improved in strength by the more
abundant consumption of milk during growth.
The experience of Dr Friend at Christ's Hospital
School, where he greatly reduced the number
of fractures among boys by giving additional
milk and substituting butter for margarine, will
be remembered in this connection. Sometimes
improvement in curative treatment in itself acts
also in a preventive way. Thus the introduction
of a better and more rapid cure of an infectious
condition will often result in the reduction of the
total incidence of the disease. The need for fever
hospitals ought indeed to be reduced greatly in
the course of the next ten years, partly by the

elimination of diphtheria, and also by the reduction in whooping cough, measles and its sequelae broncho-pneumonia and middle ear disease, which will follow the wider adoption of improved methods of prophylaxis and treatment now available. Scarlet fever has become such a mild disease, causing only 349 deaths in 95,737 cases in England and Wales during 1937, that its segregation in fever hospitals may not, in the near future, be justifiable. On the other hand, this segregation may be an important factor in the rapid decline in killing power and also in the incidence of scarlet fever.

Thus we see two forces at work affecting hospital practice—the one necessitating its increase and demanding greater hospitals, more doctors and more nurses, the other acting more slowly but, by eliminating disease, tending to lessen the demand for these services. Although it now appears as if victory has gone to the improved diagnosis and treatment factors, the future indicates the greater and greater influence of preventive medicine. Acute killing diseases of early and middle life can be expected to get less and less common and the chronic disabling diseases of old age more common. The average age of patients in hospitals will probably increase and, except for motor accidents, hospitals will become to a greater extent places for the alleviation of suffering and

(36)

for the provision of comfort for the aged rather than places where dramatic cures are performed and the sick restored to health.

From an economic standpoint and especially from the point of view of running civic and voluntary hospitals and institutions, it is clear that, only by encouraging medical research and by promptly adopting methods of preventing disease as they come to light, can the present tremendously costly system be controlled.

As for the effect of additional knowledge on the total amount of medical attention required, this latter ought to be reduced greatly, assuming that the call on the doctor's services remain at the present level for individual complaints. There will, however, be a change in the nature of his work and a greater proportion will be directed to protection against disease, and services in preventive medicine may be proportionately, but possibly not absolutely, increased. It will, for instance, almost certainly be much more the doctor's duty to protect young people against diphtheria, whooping cough and measles than to attend them suffering from these conditions. Methods of affording protection against epidemic influenza, which in the pandemic of 1918-19 killed over 10 million people, may soon be at the disposal of the doctor. Unfortunately, no method of protection against the common cold is yet in sight. Nor does there seem any immediate hope of reducing greatly the high incidence of digestive troubles with their more serious sequelae, gastric and duodenal ulcer and appendicitis. These common complaints may, however, yield to investigation at any time and it is quite evident that the general practitioner's work, as at present carried out, may be reduced greatly and even seriously from his point of view, in the near future. At the same time, the improved weapons constantly placed at his disposal by medical science must make his work more effective.

At first sight, the future of the dental surgeon seems even more precarious, for there is little doubt that knowledge of methods of building up soundly formed teeth, in well-developed jaws with good healthy gums by the proper feeding of infants and children, is definitely established. The immediate causes of caries and pyorrhoea are less understood, except in so far as they are not so likely to develop in perfectly formed teeth and gums. There can be little doubt that not many years will have passed before there will be available for parents precise knowledge as to how to produce in their children perfect teeth, relatively free from caries, but it is equally certain that many parents will not carry out these instructions. The improvement in the teeth may actually increase the amount of dental work, because it will allow the treatment of caries and other dental diseases to be more worth while than at present, when a large part of the population is edentulous at the age of thirty or forty.

The future of the public health services also is difficult to foresee. Except for the provision of centres for the medical care of children of two to five years and schemes for providing and controlling supplies of milk and other protective foods to the poor, there does not seem much reason at present for a great increase in these services. On the other hand, the need for some of the established services ought to be less in the near future. This is certainly true of fever hospitals, as shown previously. If tuberculosis maintains its downward grade of the past seventy years, the need for treatment centres and public institutions for this disease ought to have nearly disappeared by 1960. The demand for treatment centres for venereal disease will probably also decline greatly and gonorrhoea cases, fewer in number, will tend to revert to the general practitioner. There does not in fact appear to be much support for the view commonly expressed that there will be a big expansion of the public health services in the future, although it is probably true that this work will assume greater relative importance.

MEDICAL KNOWLEDGE AS THE LIMITING
FACTOR IN PUBLIC HEALTH SCHEMES

When considering problems of health and disease for this lecture, I was constantly brought up against the question of the philosophy of government which decided the particular kind of health legislation to receive attention at any time. I cannot pretend to be able to answer this question. Clearly the provision of free hospital accommodation and medical treatment for the sick poor and the provision of health insurance, whose main drawback is its limitation, are all to the good and need no justification. It is in fact almost impossible to criticise severely any particular health legislation, whether it concerns antenatal clinics, or child-welfare centres, or administrative schemes for midwifery or for the treatment of tuberculosis, venereal disease or cancer. Each scheme is bound to have some beneficial effect and the only difficulty is to understand why some of these particular schemes were chosen before, for instance, schemes for medical provision for children two to five years old or the adequate supply of milk and other protective foods to all school children or the prophylaxis against diphtheria. It is difficult to avoid the conclusion that the dominant factor in deciding health legislation has often a political rather than a scientific basis.

(40)

What I am now particularly concerned with, however, is to emphasise that any State scheme affecting health can only be as effective as medical knowledge at that time allows it to be. However large and grandiose the scheme adopted, however costly, however well administered, the limiting factor for effectiveness must be knowledge of the treatment to be practised in each particular case. If scientific knowledge is good and its application adequate, the scheme will be successful; if poor, unsuccessful. If, during the running of a scheme, research brings to light better medical knowledge, the results of the scheme improve accordingly. These statements must sound trite. Practical experience would not indicate, however, that appreciation of their truth is widespread. It is impossible to deal fully with the question here, and reference to one or two administrative schemes only will be made to demonstrate this point.

Venereal disease. The official government action against venereal disease had its origin in the Venereal Diseases Act of 1917, when treatment centres were set up throughout the country. During this period, the treatment of the two venereal diseases, syphilis and gonorrhoea, from the point of view of effecting a rapid cure, cannot be regarded as satisfactory. It is true that the discovery of Ehrlich, who introduced organic-arsenical compounds in 1910 for the treatment of

(41)

syphilis, represented a very great advance, but the complete cure of the disease by this means often extends over a period of two years. It is probable, however, that the infectivity of a patient suffering from syphilis is greatly reduced before he is completely cured. In the case of gonorrhoea, the treatment has been in the past even less satisfactory, because infectivity often remains when the patient thinks himself cured. Gonorrhoea is also not regarded with the same horror by the average patient as is syphilis, and the corresponding lack of care only makes the treatment more difficult and the spread of infection less controllable. The incidence of 'new cases' at the treatment centres throughout the country since 1925 is as follows:

	1925	1933	1934	1935	1937
(a) *Syphilis*					
Males	11,782	10,738	9,615	8,596	8,069
Females	7,385	6,029	5,838	5,565	5,165
Total	19,167	16,767	15,453	14,161	13,234
(b) *Gonorrhoea*					
Males	24,398	29,169	28,787	27,506	29,250
Females	6,120	8,583	8,199	7,732	7,787
Total	30,518	37,752	36,986	35,238	37,037

It will be seen that the incidence of syphilis has been steadily reduced from 19,167 cases in 1925 to 13,234 in 1937, whereas that of gonorrhoea has increased from 30,518 in 1925 to 37,037 in 1937, although this figure has been about stationary since 1933. Clearly the limiting factor is knowledge of methods of treating these diseases, for there can be little doubt as to the efficiency with which the medical personnel apply the knowledge available. With the discovery of a greatly improved method of treating gonorrhoea during the past year, it is almost certain that the incidence of this disease will drop rapidly in future years. As the result of intensive clinical trials during the past year, there is general agreement that 2-sulphanilyl-aminopyradine or sulfapyridine (as the Americans call it) cures over 80 per cent of patients suffering from gonorrhoea in a little over a week's treatment. This contrasts with the five or more months' treatment previously required in such cases. This discovery probably sounds the death knell of one of the scourges of civilisation. If a similar advance in the chemotherapeutic treatment of syphilis were discovered, the need for treatment centres of venereal disease would probably rapidly end.

Maternal mortality. State interest in deaths occurring in women following pregnancy and in the newly born has been shown in the Midwives Acts of 1902 and 1936. In recent years the subject has become of greater importance because the death-rate of such women did not show the decline that has been seen to occur in many other diseases. In particular, sepsis, about which so much knowledge has accumulated, continued to increase from year to year. The following figures show this fact:

Deaths ascribed to pregnancy and child-bearing

Year	Live births registered	No. of deaths	Death rates per 100,000 live births registered		
			Puerperal sepsis	Other puerperal causes	Total puerperal mortality
1912	872,737	3473	1·39	2·59	3·98
1919	692,438	3028	1·67	2·70	4·37
1925	710,582	2900	1·56	2·52	4·08
1930	648,811	2854	1·92	2·48	4·40
1934	597,642	2748	2·03	2·57	4·60
1935	598,756	2457	1·68	2·42	4·11
1936	605,292	2301	1·39	2·41	3·80
1937	—	—	0·94	2·19	3·13

These figures show that the mortality rates due to both sepsis and other causes have remained almost constant until 1936, when the last Midwives Act was introduced. It might be thought that the decline in 1936 and in 1937 was due to the new administrative scheme, and so to some extent it may be. It will be noticed, however, that the fall in death-rate is almost entirely due to the decrease in deaths from sepsis, decrease in deaths due to toxaemias of pregnancy and other causes being

(44)

very small. It may be asked whether any new advance in knowledge could account for the decreased deaths due to sepsis. There were two such great discoveries—the main one being that of Dr Leonard Colebrook, who showed that prontosil and other sulphanilamide compounds had a curative action in puerperal sepsis and was able to bring the death-rate of women suffering from this disease at Queen Charlotte's Hospital from an average figure of 22 per cent down to between 4 and 5 per cent by this treatment. The second discovery was the establishment of the fact that many of the most serious cases of puerperal sepsis owed their infection to streptococci conveyed to the birth canal from the respiratory tract of the medical or nursing attendants. This observation cleared up a difficulty which has long confronted medical men, namely, that in spite of all aseptic and antiseptic precautions of modern times, the incidence and mortality of puerperal sepsis have remained unlowered. It is now evident that, if medical and nursing attendants take the same precautions in preventing infection from their breath gaining access to women in childbirth as they take in the care of their hands, serious cases of puerperal septicaemia will be substantially diminished. When such infections take place, we have now the second line of defence, previously mentioned, namely, a powerful curative remedy. Here again, therefore, it can be predicted that the fall in incidence of deaths due to puerperal sepsis will continue. The day will no doubt arrive when another advance in knowledge will reveal the cause and methods of prevention of the other large cause of death in childbirth, viz. the toxaemias of pregnancy. But in this case also it will be the discovery that matters, although it is also true that the machinery of the Midwives Act will allow the discovery to be used to good advantage.

The treatment of cancer. In recent months we have seen the passage of the Cancer Act through Parliament, an Act which provides increased facilities for the treatment of this disease. There are now 74,000 deaths annually in this country due to cancer, a number which is increasing, largely because the average age of the people is rising. State action in this matter was taken mainly because of alarm at the increasing incidence, and not because of any large increase in proportion of permanent cures that can be expected from the increased facilities for treatment as at present practised. In other words, the medical scientist, using benefits in terms of life as his criterion, would not at the present time have encouraged the setting up of this scheme in priority to other possible public actions affecting health. The reason for this is simply that the present methods of treating cancer, except in certain cases, are not good enough to lead to the expectation of great saving of life, even when more extensively used.

The whole future of this disease depends upon increased knowledge and improved methods of combating it, which such knowledge will ensure. Even the best of the present methods of treatment by radium and X-rays could be greatly improved by research. Both of these methods of radiation are powerful instruments for harm if not properly used, and it will require a great effort to see that the optimum conditions are adopted in the treatment centres. Success of the Cancer Act in the future almost certainly lies with improvement in radiological methods of treatment by X-rays and radium and the opening up of new lines of attack, which can only be developed by more knowledge of the fundamental nature of cancer. To the biological investigator, cancer is the most enigmatical problem of all and, until this enigma is solved, there seems but little likelihood of the treatment of the disease becoming really effective and curative.

No better instance could be given of the limiting factor of knowledge in a State enterprise for tackling a specific problem of disease. During the past year, the importance of the cancer problem has been equally recognised by the Government of the United States of America, but the method of dealing with the situation has been different. Instead of embarking upon a State scheme for treating cancer, they have set aside large sums of money for cancer research and have inaugurated the National Cancer Institute. It is fortunate that we in this country shall be able to share in the fruits of this action for stimulating the acquisition of knowledge, but it is less pleasant to think that they, on their part, may not be able to benefit to the same extent by our own particular Government scheme for dealing with this problem.

The whole position of State action in health matters wants clarifying. Sentiment and 'public appeal', associated with particular lines of action, ought to be eliminated and each proposition ought to be considered only from the point of view of results to be expected from administrative schemes in terms of saving life and affording increased efficiency to individuals. Administrative and advisory bodies concerned with matters of health must also make up their minds what they want, which of the many problems of public health ought to receive priority and which problems can be regarded, on the basis of present knowledge, as likely to yield rapidly and successfully to attack. On general lines a decision ought to be taken as to whether the prime object is to save child and early life and allow citizens to grow up with optimum physical and mental health or to eliminate disease of elderly people and extend life at that end of the scale.

Everybody will agree that once a decision has been taken by Government to deal with a problem of ill-health, it is not sufficient to set up the necessary administrative organisation, but every effort must be made, by giving facilities for research, to see that the best brains available are directed to the discovery of improved medical methods for dealing with the situation. At the present moment this applies specially to the cancer problem.

HEALTH, FERTILITY AND POPULATIONS

It has already been stressed that, apart from raising the standards of health and physique, the outstanding effect of medical science in the present century has been to reduce the incidence of or to eliminate the main fatal diseases of early and adult life. Whereas 15,619 children aged one to five years out of each million living at this age in 1911–14 died, this figure in 1935 was 5075 and it is still diminishing. There has also been an appreciable reduction in rates of mortality at older ages, including early manhood and middle life, but these reductions are not so spectacular as in the first years of life. There is no evidence that rates of mortality among the aged, i.e. over seventy years, are decreasing. On account of these changes, expectation of life has increased considerably in recent years as the following figures, kindly provided by Professor Greenwood, show:

Approximate expectation of life in years

		0	5	10	45
1871–80	Male	41·35	50·87	47·60	22·07
	Female	44·62	53·08	49·76	24·06
1891–1900	Male	44·13	53·50	49·63	22·20
	Female	47·77	55·79	51·97	24·20
1910–12	Male	51·50	57·14	53·91	23·92
	Female	55·35	59·94	55·91	26·34
1923–25	Male	56·90	59·40	54·60	25·30
	Female	60·60	62·20	58·00	27·70
1930–32	Male	58·74	60·11	55·79	25·51
	Female	62·88	63·24	58·87	28·30
1935–37	Male	60·17	60·73	56·41	25·53
(approximate, Snow's method)	Female	64·35	64·06	59·70	28·59

It will be seen that from the end of the last
century to the present day, the expectation of life
of those newly born has increased 16 years in the
case of males and over 16½ years in females, and
that boys born now can expect to reach the age of
60 years and girls 64 years. A similar change has
taken place in America as the following figures,
provided by the Metropolitan Life Insurance Com-
pany of New York, show. At the age of ten the
expectation of life of white males in 1911–12 was
45·61 years, that of white females 50·66. By 1935
the comparable figures were 53·68 for white males
and 57·65 for white females. Thus between the
years 1912 and 1935 white males in America at

age ten added 8·07 years and white females 6·99 years to their life span.

Partly due to, this lengthening of life of the average individual and partly to the reduction in birth rate that has been a prominent feature in this and many other countries in recent years, the proportionate number of old people in the population has gone steadily up and promises to continue to do so. In 1911, there were 297 people over seventy in every 10,000 of the population: in 1935 this figure had increased to 467. In 1911 there were 1158 over fifty-five years old in 10,000 of the population: in 1935 this figure was 1810.

From a sociological standpoint the diminution in the birth rate is of much greater significance than the increased length of life, especially as we have seen that mortality rates have not been lowered recently for people over seventy. As the reduction in childbirth does not seem to be primarily a medical problem, I shall not discuss the subject here. Even if medical science advanced to the extent of being able to save all the infants born, so that they lived through the full average span of life, it would make but little difference to the sociological problem that has to be faced. All that medical science can do is to assure women that at no stage in the world's history has it been possible for them to bear children with less detriment to themselves, with greater certainty of healthy babies and with more assurance that these babies will ultimately attain a good age with better standards of physique and general health than at earlier times. It is indeed nature's grimmest joke that medical science is establishing the optimum conditions for safe birth and healthy existence just at the time when fewer and fewer babies are born.

Whatever may be the cause or causes of the present situation the two fundamental conditions of reversing the process and of obtaining a greater birth rate are (1) earlier marriage, and (2) a desire for larger families. Either condition alone may not solve the problem, as it may well be that modern conditions of life in this country make people sterile at an earlier age than in former years. The situation can be stated in a few words. There were nearly a million less children (ages 0–14) at the census of 1931 than at the census of 1921: between 1931 and 1937 there has been a further fall of nearly 600,000. At present 25 per cent more babies must be born to maintain the population of the country, but this figure will rapidly rise if the decline in birth rate continues.

Many of the social and economic implications of these modern developments in population have been pointed out by others. Geneticists and psychologists have informed us that reduction in size of families is producing lower average intelligence in the country. It has also been shown by economists that a lowered birth rate will not solve the unemployment problem and indeed will make it worse. On the other hand, the burden of doing the work of the country and of maintaining a population of older people will fall on fewer young people. The rapidly increasing members of the community over sixty years of age will have to be maintained by an even more rapidly diminishing number of workers under fifty, who in addition, will have to maintain all the social services at their present or at a higher level as well as earn the interest on the enormous national debt.

If, therefore, there is truth in the statement that married people are refusing to have children because of their desire to raise the standard of life for themselves and their families, they are living in a fool's paradise and laying up for themselves and their children a hard future. The present discussions about increased leisure can have little or no meaning, in view of the falling birth rate and prolonged life of the individual. Indeed the indications are all to the contrary and, in spite of the advances in production by machinery and the discoveries of agriculture, there can be little doubt that, assuming the continuance of the existing economic and social system, the present standards of living will only be maintained in the future by harder and more prolonged efforts of the working population.

It may be well to remember in this connection also that medical science has not yet seriously tackled the problems of degenerative disease and old age. There is no reason whatever why solutions or partial solutions to these problems should not be obtained, as has been so often the case with other problems of life. Already there is good experimental evidence that the life span of animals can be lengthened by diet, especially by increasing the amount of milk consumed. In the case of male rats the average life span was increased from 651 to 705 days by this means (H. C. Sherman and H. L. Campbell, *J. Nutrition*, 1935, x, 363). In other experiments it was shown that the life span of animals could be increased by reducing the total intake of a good diet and retarding the rate of growth. In these experiments also it was the males that were affected, their life span being increased from 483 to 820 days, that of the females remaining constant at about 800 days (C. M. McCay, M. F. Crowell and L. A. Maynard, *J. Nutrition*, 1935, x, 63).

Whereas it is probable that these effects of diet might well apply to man, it must be pointed out that the experimental results, interesting as they are, do not touch the essential problem of old age, namely, the degenerative changes in the tissues that take place. These rats, as they aged, however they were fed, developed many of the usual cardiovascular degenerative changes and other changes such as blindness. Thus, although proper feeding, both as to quantity and quality of food, may well extend the life span of man, the main problem of old age is not solely one of nutrition but of some other type, such as the inability of the cells to build up specific chemical substances or to maintain the effective chemical balance of early life. This does not make the problem of old age insoluble but only shifts its solution to another direction, and anybody who is familiar with the modern amazing discoveries of hormone physiology will not regard such a problem as beyond man's ability to solve. Nothing seems impossible to medical research nowadays, and the mere fact that a problem of physiology or pathology can be clearly formulated in the human mind indicates that it may be solved to the extent that human control of the phenomenon can be partially or completely obtained. This may well happen in the case of old age.

Suppose by medical research man did in fact discover means of deferring death by finding out and controlling the changes of old age, would such discoveries be applied to human life? It is impossible to be sure on this point. If, for instance, it were now possible, as it probably is, to say categorically that the average human span of life could be immediately increased, say five years, by the general consumption of a pint or a quart of milk a day, by moderation in other foods and abstinence from smoking and excessive consumption of alcoholic beverages, would such teaching affect the average individual? Probably not. Most men would answer, 'Keep your milk and your extra five years of life, and we will keep our good feeding, our tobacco and our alcohol'. Men indeed seem often to have but little interest in length of life in itself, but they do have an intense desire to retain those qualities and amenities of life which give them great pleasure. If, therefore, lengthening the span of life involved doing or experiencing something not entirely agreeable or restricting their pleasures over a long period of time, it is not likely to be generally adopted. But we can never be certain, and sociologists and economists, already worried as they are about the population question, with the diminishing birth rate and greater proportion of old people, must not exclude from their calculations the possibility that medical science will ultimately, and in the not distant future, get some controlling influence over old age. We can only hope that, if the effects of age are to be studied, some success will also be obtained in elucidating the chemical processes actually responsible for these degenerative changes. By such knowledge only will it be possible to defer the signs and symptoms of age and to lengthen the active period of the lives of men and women. If it should happen that the first effect of medical research is to increase the span of life of the average healthy adult from the proverbial threescore years and ten to fourscore years and ten, in such a way that the last twenty years of life are accompanied by mental degeneration and physical decrepitude, the outlook is indeed gloomy.

It will be clear then that, so far as its beneficial effect on population in this country is concerned, medical science has almost shot its bolt, except possibly that it may extend the fertility period of women desirous of bearing children. It is the factor mainly responsible for the increase in number of people in England and Wales from 14,000,000 in 1840 to 41,000,000 in 1937. Only qualitatively in terms of standards of health and physique, where medical science has already done so much, has it still a big contribution to make.

MEDICAL SCIENCE AND TROPICAL COUNTRIES

This, however, is not the case in our colonial territories, especially those inhabited largely by native races. Knowledge, bringing control of tropical diseases, has increased enormously in recent years, and there is every evidence that the British Government intends to press forward with the application of this knowledge for the benefit of

(57)

native races. We can expect, therefore, in the near future a repetition in colonial territories of what has happened in this country in the past hundred years. The native populations will increase greatly and the standards of physique and health will be raised. The limiting factor in these changes will not be knowledge of tropical disease or lack of desire to apply such knowledge but the success obtained in each country in producing sufficient food for the growing population. If, for instance, India cannot grow or purchase sufficient food for its rapidly increasing population, nothing that good administration or medical science can do will prevent a social disaster. Advances in agricultural production must therefore keep pace with population changes and the foods produced must be considered, not only from the point of view of energy but from that of modern nutritional requirements in relation to health and physique. It may be some consolation to the agriculturist to know that advances in knowledge of human health will be generally applicable to animal life.

Much social and economic trouble will be prevented if these developments are foreseen as a whole and plans made for meeting them now. With the rise in standards of living that will follow the best type of administrative action, the high fertility rates now found in native races will undoubtedly diminish, as they have done in this country, and the balance of numbers will tend to be restored. There are great troubles ahead and many people would feel happier about the future of native races if more men with scientific training and outlook, especially on the biological side, held the important administrative posts in colonial countries. There can be but little doubt that most of the political, social and economic difficulties in tropical countries are, and will continue to be, biological in nature, and the sooner this fact is recognised the sooner will these difficulties be controlled or dispersed. There are some people who recognise the difficulties of the future, and some of these look with disfavour at the extension of medical knowledge and its application to native people. Having put our hands to the plough, however, there can be no turning back, and we can only pray that there is sufficient wisdom left among us to use the fruits of science properly.

There are many other problems, not mentioned in this lecture, which ought to be discussed. The geneticist and his subject have not received consideration because he is still collecting his data but, in course of time, the facts he is collecting will have to be faced by our administrators. In particular, the importance of mental disorder, both from the genetic and other points of view, will demand much greater attention. At present success has been mainly attained in keeping the mentally defective physically healthy and extending their lives, and the enormous burden on the country has been thereby increased. Only by increasing knowledge of the cause, finding methods of prevention and cure of mental disorder, can any hope be based for alleviating or mastering the present situation.

CONCLUSION

It will probably be agreed that medical science has had and will continue to have a very great effect on the life of the community. Every person, in whatever capacity, must be influenced. The individual is guaranteed better health and physical development and longer life, the woman is given the promise of easier childbirth, more certain survival of her offspring and less wasted effort in bringing up her family; the doctor's total work may be reduced but it will be more effective; the State will have at its disposal a finer race of people. This new knowledge, however, brings to each added duties and responsibilities, for increased benefits can only be obtained by appreciating it and making use of it. If, indeed, the past is any criterion, the adoption of the teachings of medical science will greatly lag behind the new discoveries. The extent of this lag will depend on medical leadership, on doctors themselves, on public health authorities, and on the intelligence of the public.

As regards medical men, the rate of increase in knowledge in medicine is so great that only by an effort can the average doctor keep up to date. On the other hand, medical literature is as exciting nowadays as any in the world, and the doctor who does not keep pace with discovery must be both unimaginative and out of his proper vocation. Fortunately each major discovery allows the jettying of much previous knowledge, so that the total effect brings little or no increased burden to the practitioner. The rapidity of medical advance must be paralleled by an equal alertness on the part of the doctor.

The State also must make up its mind how best to use new knowledge. Does it intend to use that for the prevention at least as rapidly as that for the cure of disease? Does it wish to encourage the development of good health and physique in the young, rather than reduce disease and extend life of the aged? Does it wish its actions to be determined by the fruitfulness of established knowledge, or does it prefer to back schemes where knowledge is undeveloped and profit of action, in terms of life and health, small? There are also important problems of public health in which action is almost completely frustrated by vested interests. This subject calls for urgent consideration by the State. Finally, the State will also have to decide, especially if it continues to provide increased facilities for health, to what extent the individual, and especially the parent, can wilfully avoid making use of these facilities and thereby allow the development of ill-health. The days of Erewhon may not be far distant.

Medical science and its instrument, medical research, have indeed justified themselves. For every problem—social and economic—raised in this lecture, the only solution is more knowledge and more wisdom to use this knowledge. There is no limit to the amount of knowledge to be gained, if the medical scientist is given the opportunities and facilities for his work. Would that the same could be said about the wisdom necessary to make the best use of this knowledge!

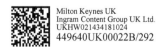

Milton Keynes UK
Ingram Content Group UK Ltd.
UKHW021434181024
449640UK00022B/292